WORKING WITH THE
MENTALLY ILL

Stories That Will Make You Smile,

Laugh, and Maybe Cry

WORKING WITH THE MENTALLY ILL

Stories That Will Make You Smile,

Laugh, and Maybe Cry

Pat Beattie

Library of Congress Control Number:		2009911061
ISBN:	Hardcover	978-1-4500-1979-8
	Softcover	978-1-4415-9150-0

This book was printed in the United States of America.

To order additional copies of this book, contact:
Xlibris Corporation
1-888-795-4274
www.Xlibris.com
Orders@Xlibris.com
70734

Contents

This book is dedicated in loving memory of my parents, who always urged me to write.

And to Denise and Karen, the two best friends anyone could have.

Preface

I had several reasons for wanting to write this book. First and foremost, I want to help educate members of our society about people who suffer from mental illness. I believe there is a misconception that the only people who have mental health problems are those who are uneducated, poor, come from broken homes, abuse drugs or alcohol, or even in some way brought their illness on themselves. This could not be further from the truth. As you read the stories of the various characters in this book, you will see that developing a mental illness can happen to anyone at any time in their life. No one is immune, and that is a particularly scary and sobering thought. If you are the type of person who makes fun of mentally ill people, think they have no feelings or cannot tell you are uncomfortable around them, or think they should all be locked up and have the key thrown away, consider this, it could one day be you or someone you care about on the receiving end of these behaviors and ideas based totally on ignorance of the topic. We tend to fear the unknown and most people aren't familiar with anyone who has a severe mental illness. I hope by reading about some of the patients I have known through the years you will realize they are not monsters but human beings who for the most part come from families who love and care about them and are also struggling because of their illness.

I also would hope that anyone interested in entering the mental health profession would read this book. It may help you decide whether or not to pursue a career in this field. It's definitely not for everyone. Many well intentioned people have tried to work with the mentally ill and found it to be too frustrating, depressing, and at times dangerous. You aren't going to be able to "cure" most of these people. You are, at best, only going to be able to help them better manage their illness and hopefully live happier and more productive lives.

I learned a great deal from the patients and inmates I had contact with throughout the years. Most important, you are not going to like all of your patients. This is just part of being human. You don't like everyone you meet in the community so why should you feel you have to like all of the patients you encounter. Just remember, even though you may not like them, you must treat them with dignity and respect. This can be difficult when a patient is spitting at you or trying to physically harm you, but you have got to keep yourself under control. If you can't do this, you need to find another occupation.

Many of the patients may be more educated or come from a higher socio-economic background than you. Education and social status has nothing to do with whether or not a person develops a mental illness.

Even though some patients may have done unacceptable things in the community or committed heinous crimes you cannot judge them. Frequently when the patient committed his/her crime they were not receiving any care for their mental illness. After being placed on medication and having the medication take effect, many of these people are actually very nice people and are horrified by the crime they committed. Unfortunately, once their legal issues are resolved and they are back out in the community, there is often a lack of support system available to them. Many stop taking their medications and in turn regress and once again find themselves in need of hospitalization or involved in the legal system for committing another crime. For many, it's a never-ending cycle of legal issues, hospitalizations, and suffering. We definitely need a better system to support people with mental illnesses.

De-institutionalization began in the 1970's and has continued. Many institutions were over-crowded, poorly run, and many patients were abused by unscrupulous staff. This is a sad fact. However, many patients also flourished in institutional settings. They had structure in their lives, learned skills, had friends, and were taken care of by staff that genuinely cared about them. Many staff members worked at institutions for over 10 years and became like family to the patients. When the patients were moved into new settings without familiar staff it caused some to regress. While many patients released to community settings have done well, others have not been as fortunate. Without structure and support, many were victimized and taken advantage of by predators in the community. If and when they realize they've been victimized, they are often hesitant to seek help for fear of being re-hospitalized because they did something wrong.

Money is one of the biggest issues in the care of people with mental illness. Government wants out of the mental health business due to the rising costs. Yet, are they really saving money? Closing mental institutions seems to have resulted in building more prisons, which are just another form of institutions. Prisons are not equipped to deal with inmates with serious mental health issues and the patient/inmate is often further victimized.

The characters in this book are based on patients and inmates I had the opportunity to work with during my career. Names as well as some details in their stories have been changed to protect their privacy.

I hope you will read their stories and try to imagine what their lives must be like. Many had mental problems from birth, but many developed their illnesses later in life. Let this serve as a reminder that none of us should ever take our mental health for granted.

Pat Beattie

MEET: The Author

I began working for the Department of Public Welfare at a residential facility for mentally retarded individuals in 1973. It was my senior year in high school and it was part of a work-study program. We could work half the day at a job and then went to school for our core classes the other half of the day. We were supposed to be working in fields that we thought would be of interest to us when choosing a career. I had always liked helping people and thought working with the retarded would be interesting. When I began working for the state, I had no idea I would remain in its employ for 34 years. Throughout my service I worked at four state hospitals and two prisons. I started my career as a Mental Retardation Aide Trainee and worked my way into the Physical Therapy Department as a Physical Therapy Aide II. When I left that particular hospital due to its pending closing, I became a Psychiatric Security Aide in the forensic unit of another state hospital. The forensic unit is different from the civil section of the state hospital because it houses men and women who are either in jail or prison awaiting trial or serving their sentences and due to behavior at those facilities are court ordered to be admitted to the forensic unit of the state hospital for evaluation and/or treatment. It is similar to a mini-prison and the staff is similar to corrections officers only they are taught to interact with the prisoner/patient in a therapeutic manner. Not all state hospitals have forensic units, in fact most do not. At the time, they had only male patients at the forensic unit I was hired to work at, but were hiring female staff to train for a year prior to opening their first female unit. I worked in the forensic unit for approximately six years before transferring to the civil section of the hospital (those patients who do not have legal issues) into the Occupational Therapy Department as a Therapeutic Activities Worker. After five years I transferred to a different state hospital due to downsizing. I worked in the Recreation Department there for six months when I was once again transferred due to downsizing. At the last state hospital, I was again in the Recreation Department. I stayed there for almost two years but could see the writing on the wall as all state hospitals were either being closed or severely downsized.

I decided to take the civil service test for an Activities position in the Department of Corrections. There were two state prisons within driving distance of my home. I have to admit, when I got the notice for an interview at the maximum security prison (for male prisoners) closest to my home, I was very hesitant. In fact, I initially replied that I was not available for the job. However, the Human Resources person called me at home and convinced me just to come for the interview and then see where things led. I interviewed and was selected for the position of Activities Specialist. I would be the only female working in a department along with eight men in a prison with 3200 male prisoners. Most of these men were serving life sentences and would never be getting out of prison. This was bound to be an experience! I worked at that particular prison for eight years, eventually working my way up to Correctional Activities Manager I. I left to become the Correctional Activities Manager II at a medium security prison that dealt mainly with offenders who had drug and alcohol problems. Most of these men had less than two years left on their sentences and were being prepared to return to life in the community. I retired from that position in June of 2007.

Throughout my time in state service, I have had the pleasure of working with many fine people and of course some not so fine ones as well. I prefer to remember the good ones and those who helped me along the way. To them I will always be grateful.

I also had the privilege of meeting some memorable individuals who had the misfortune of suffering from mental retardation and/or serious mental illness as well as many interesting men who reside within the confines of prison walls. While I may not have liked all of the patients and prisoners I came in contact with, and believe me, I didn't, I believe I learned something from each and every one of them. I hope I was able to teach them something as well.

Many people have asked me over the years, "How can you work at a place like that?" or "How can you work with "those people?" I really don't have an answer. I just always tried to remember these people all had lives before becoming patients and/or prisoners. Many of them have families who love them and many were quite productive in society before their circumstances changed. Believe it or not, they all have feelings too, despite what they may want you to think. Many of them have developed a hardened outer layer in order to survive in a world you or I cannot imagine. But, deep down, they still have feelings, for after all, they are human beings. I've found that in most cases, if you treat someone with dignity and respect, they will treat you with dignity and respect.

One of the biggest lessons I learned is just because a person has a mental illness, do not make the mistake of thinking they're stupid. Many individuals with mental illness are very intelligent and worked at good jobs prior to becoming ill. I've seen patients come from all walks of life, nurses, artists, laborers, business people, just to name a few. These people were making a good living and providing for their families before their various illnesses caused them to be hospitalized. The good news is that if they can become stabilized on medication, many will be able to return to their former lives and once again be productive members of the community and responsible family members. I would often supervise the visiting room and at times it could be heartbreaking to see the suffering the family members were going through along with the patient.

12

Another lesson I learned is that patients generally remember what was said or done to them when they were sick. I always assumed since they were in a psychotic state or not in touch with reality that they didn't know what was going on around them. That is not the case. There was a young man named Chris, who had been extremely psychotic when he was brought to the forensic unit. He had auditory and visual hallucinations and it took several months before he was stabilized and able to be sent back to the county jail. The night before he left, he said goodbye to me and said, "You know, you were the only one who would talk to me when I was sick. The others just kept away from me or made fun of me." I also know of patients who have attacked staff once they were considered more stable because of something the staff person said or did to them when they were very sick. So, keep this in mind if you have chosen the mental health field as a career. Another thing I always tried to remember was that patient could be me or one of my family members. How would I want to be treated or have my family member treated? Hopefully, that will put it in perspective for you.

Many patients are extremely delusional when they enter the hospital. As staff, we have always been taught no to feed into their delusions. While I agree with that to some degree, I will argue that there are times when it's not such a bad thing to go along with them. If a patient is admitted to your unit and honestly believes she is the Queen of England you are not going to change her mind right away. Whenever a patient is admitted, they have to be interviewed by the psychiatric aide staff on the unit to have their vital signs taken, notations are made for any visible scars or tattoos, and other important information. One of the questions we would ask was, "How do you wish to be addressed?" Some would say, "Mary" or "Mr. Jones." Others would give answers relating to their delusions, such as, "Your Majesty" or Queen Linda." If you want to develop a therapeutic rapport with this patient, calling her Mary (if that is her real name) is only going to upset her and possible get you hurt if she becomes agitated. If you want her to take her medication, take a shower, or go to meals, it is much easier to say, "Queen Linda, it's time for medication." She is more likely to cooperate if you call her what she wants to be called at this time. I know that many of the professionals I have worked with will disagree with this, but generally, they are not the ones working with the patients for 8 hours at a time and actually seeing how they respond and interact with others. I had a patient one time that wanted to be called "Bob" when she first came in as she was convinced she was a male. After about 2 weeks, I went to call her for medication, saying, "Bob, it's time for meds." She promptly looked at me and said, "My name isn't Bob, I'm Beth." The medication had started to work and she was coming out of her delusional state. After that she would respond to her given name. I don't see the harm in calling them Queen Linda or Mr. President if that is going to help them remain calm and lead to them being more cooperative with staff. They are already agitated enough simply by being in the hospital and at times facing legal issues, why add to or increase their agitation at this time.

Working with prisoners was another thing many of my family and friends couldn't understand. I tried to explain that whatever the inmate did that had landed him in prison had nothing to do with me. He was there to serve his time. Working in the Activities Department made the job easier since activities are considered a privilege and if the prisoner acts out he will lose the privilege of participating in sports, music, or other things most of the men look forward to. They have so few privileges as it is, they don't want to lose any.

The Activities staff members in the prisons are often looked down on by many of the Correctional Officers. We're called "Inmate Lovers" because we provide recreational activities for those who have committed some very serious, and at times, heinous crimes. Whenever a new class of Correctional Officers came through the Activities Department on their orientation, I would stress to them that inmates who were involved in activities are generally too busy or too tired to be sitting around conjuring up ways to create havoc for the officers. Activities provide an outlet for them to release pent up energy in an acceptable manner. Sports provide an opportunity for the inmate to learn to work as a team member and share responsibility. These are lessons most of us learn as children, but many of these men were already out on the streets hustling for a buck when they were children.

Many of the men I worked with at the prisons were serving life terms. They are never getting out of prison. When they are processed into the facility they are asked where they want their body to go when they die. For many of them, that's the first time they realize what a life sentence really means. I've known inmates who have put in between 25 and 35 years. I don't know how they do it. I doubt I would be strong enough to survive that many years in that type of environment. Try to imagine what it would be like to live in an 8 by 10 foot cell. Now consider that you could also be sharing that small space with a "cellie" who you may not like, or who may have poor hygiene, or other negative traits. Go into your bathroom at home, close the door, and think what it would be like to live in there. The only difference is instead of a bathtub, you would have a bunk. Cells have a bunk, toilet, sink, and writing desk. That's all. Inmates participate in a variety of activities to avoid being in their cells. Hopefully while participating in the activities they are able to learn something constructive.

With all of this being said, I would now like you to read about some of the most interesting people I've ever met.

MEET: Jasmine

When I first met Jasmine she was in her mid twenties. Over the six year period I worked in the forensic unit at the state hospital, Jasmine was admitted and discharged four times.

Jasmine has been diagnosed as mildly mentally retarded and also suffers from mental illness. Though somewhat functional when she is in the community, she often makes poor decisions which result in her numerous arrests on charges of prostitution, petty theft, assault, etc. Jasmine has little support from her family as her mother appears to have some mental problems of her own and is raising Jasmine's teenage daughter. The daughter writes to Jasmine sporadically and appears to be a good student. Jasmine will frequently call home but her collect calls are generally refused, more for financial reasons than anything else. Her mother has sent her a brief letter and $5.00 once or twice in the years I knew her.

The first time Jasmine was admitted to the forensic unit she had been serving time in the county jail and was simply too disruptive for them to handle. She would alternate between being cooperative and totally out of control. She could be physically aggressive and frequently had hallucinations and heard voices. She could become very manic and silly and quickly change to angry and sobbing. She was frequently combative with staff and other patients and would strike out in response to her delusional thinking. Due to her many years of surviving in the streets of Philadelphia, she was an excellent fighter. She caused several staff members to be sent for medical attention during her various admissions. She was placed on medication which helped to a degree but when she would be discharged either back to the county jail and from there into the community, Jasmine would stop taking her medication and resort to using street drugs which would lead to her being arrested again and the cycle would continue.

On one admission it was determined that Jasmine was pregnant. Therefore, she could not be placed on any psychotropic medications. We all knew it was going to be a long, long summer. We did our best to keep Jasmine engaged in activities to enable her to focus her attention on constructive things instead of her hallucinations and, all things considered, she did pretty well.

Quite often, police press charges against the mentally ill in order to have them sent to a forensic unit for evaluation and treatment. Many of these individuals are not competent to stand trial at first but with the proper medication and various therapies, often become competent and are able to resolve their legal issues. However, this time, due to being pregnant, and unable to be placed on medication, Jasmine was basically being protected from herself and others. There was no way she was going to be able to focus on her legal issues and cooperate with her attorney without medication. In addition to her legal situation, decisions had to be made regarding the baby. Jasmine's mother was contacted and told the social worker there was no way she would take a second child into her home. She had limited income and was already caring for Jasmine's daughter. Jasmine was furious with her mother regarding this decision, but her mother remained steadfast. After much counseling, which at times was difficult due to Jasmine's frame of mind, she decided to place the baby in foster care until her legal issues could be resolved. She had hopes of taking the baby to live with her once she was released, but this never happened. The foster parents adopted Jasmine's son and gave social services frequent reports on his health and progress so Jasmine could be assured she had made the right decision.

The last time I saw Jasmine was when she was once again admitted from the county jail. This time she had been charged with going into a house and stealing a radio. The owner came home while this was in progress and called police. Jasmine had once again stopped taking her medications and was aggressive, hallucinating, and out of control. She was incompetent to stand trial on the charges and was hospitalized for treatment. Jasmine was now almost 30 years old. During this admission it was discovered she was diabetic and had to be placed on insulin. She was incapable of administering her own insulin despite the many classes the nursing staff involved her in. However, with the medication being given to her by the nurses, her diabetes was brought under control. Interestingly, once this was controlled, her behavior also improved. While she still had hallucinations and delusional ideas, she was much less aggressive and more cooperative with treatment. Unfortunately, she remained incompetent to stand trial. She probably served more time in the forensic unit trying to become competent to stand trial than she would have if found guilty of the charges. Eventually, the charges were dropped and she was transferred into the civil section of the hospital where she would be able to earn privileges and more freedom.

Despite being on the receiving end of several of Jasmine's physical assaults, she was one of my favorite patients. When her behavior was under control and she would talk about her daughter, you could see how proud she was of her. You could also see the hurt in her eyes when her mother refused her phone calls or wouldn't come to visit. Between being mildly retarded and mental illness, she had been dealt a double whammy in life and was doing her best to get by.

MEET: Angel Girl

Angel Girl came to the forensic unit of the hospital from the county jail. She had been charged with trespassing on private property. While in the county jail she was observed to be depressed and possibly suicidal, although she denied being so.

Angel Girl was a Puerto Rican girl in her mid twenties. She was tall and thin and wore her hair in two braided pigtails. She appeared very child-like and innocent. Generally she only spoke when spoken to and was cooperative with the unit's routine. It would have been easy to overlook her as she didn't cause problems. With a unit capacity of 25 females the squeaky wheels definitely get the grease.

For some reason, Angel Girl became my shadow when I was on duty. She would help me with whatever chore I might be doing, from passing out clean linens to cleaning up the shower room. In the early evening between dinner and bedtime, she would generally sit with me in the dayhall, watching TV, playing cards, or simply sitting quietly. Staff often wondered why she had been sent to the hospital as she didn't seem particularly depressed or suicidal. She was just very quiet and seemed somewhat naïve for her age. She would answer questions realistically and seemed to enjoy observing the daily routine of the unit and the antics of some of the other patients.

One evening while waiting for medications to be given out, Angel Girl began a conversation with me I will never forget. She told me about the angels that came to her room each night and how they would talk to her and tell her what to do. While I was shocked to hear her talk like this, I couldn't let on. I wanted her to feel she could confide in me and trust me. She talked for almost an hour about the angels while I just listened. I didn't confirm or deny their existence as it would've done no good. She knew they were real. Over time, she would occasionally talk to me further about the angels. She seemed to feel special that they came to her and I think this gave her a sense of peace. She never spoke to the psychiatrist or nurses about the angels, although I noted the information in her chart so they would know there was more going on with her than what we initially thought. She remained cooperative and eventually went to court where her charges were dropped.

Once charges are dropped or a person completes their sentence, they can no longer stay in the forensic unit. Most of the time they are transferred to one of the units in the civil section where they receive further treatment and are hopefully discharged when they become stable. Angel Girl was transferred to one of the units where she was able to earn privileges to go on grounds by herself and eventually she earned the privilege to go out for the day with her boyfriend. The boyfriend came to pick her up in the morning and was supposed to have her back by 4:00 p.m. Four o'clock came and went without her return. Attempts were made to contact the boyfriend, but without success. She was listed as AWOL but since she had no criminal charges at that time, she was not aggressively pursued. Two days later we found out that Angel Girl had jumped in front of a train and was killed. Apparently, her boyfriend after picking her up and having sex with her didn't feel like driving her back to the hospital so he just abandoned her in the city. She had no money and didn't know how to get back to the hospital. Somehow, she ended up at the train station and I would be willing to bet the angels told her to get on the train as it was coming into the station. What I found most infuriating about this is the fact the boyfriend was never charged with any wrongdoing. I will always feel that he caused her death and should have been charged with involuntary manslaughter at the very least. I hope Angel Girl is at peace with the other angels now.

MEET: Roberta

There was a lobby area where the psychiatric security aides would gather before starting their shifts. It was a place to exchange gossip, talk with staff from other units, and simply spend a little time with others who would be facing an 8 hour shift where almost anything could, and did happen. The PSA's were a pretty tight group and realized that you were dependent on one another if something went down. These were the people who "had your back."

The lobby was where I first heard about Roberta. She had been brought in on the day shift and apparently her arrival was rather spectacular. She had several policemen and women accompanying her, which was unusual as prisoners are usually brought by the county sheriffs. But the most talked about aspect of her arrival was her appearance. She was approximately 6'2" and weighed about 210 lbs. and upon her arrival was wearing only a bed sheet to keep her covered and her hands were chained to a belt at her waist and her legs were shackled at the ankles. She was considered very dangerous and had injured several policemen during her arrest. She was in an extremely psychotic state and it was determined that she should be placed in 4 point restraints for her own safety as well as the safety of others. When a patient was placed in 4 point restraints they were placed in a bed and had their wrists and ankles shackled to the bed with leather restraints. They were placed in a room that had the door open and had a PSA (Psychiatric Security Aide) within arms' length and watching them at all times. This is known as 1:1 observation.

As it was change of shift and there were two shifts of staff available it was decided Roberta would be taken from the bed and allowed to use the bathroom with only her hand shackled to a belt at her waist. When lying in the bed, I didn't think Roberta looked as big as she had been described. I changed my mind very quickly when we got her into a standing position. Not only was she every bit of 6'2", she had very bushy, unkempt hair that made her appear even taller! She was also very psychotic and obviously paranoid which can be a recipe for disaster. Fortunately, Roberta appeared to realize there were many more of us than there was of her and cooperated with using the bathroom and returning to the bed where she was once again placed in 4 points.

Due to her psychotic state of mind, Roberta remained in restraints for several days. As her medication began to take effect and she became less psychotic the restraints were gradually reduced and she was able to be released from all restraints and join the other patients on the unit. Once stabilized, Roberta was one of the more cooperative patients and even earned the privilege of being the paid janitor on the unit.

Roberta's legal problems began when she and her "husband" went on a drinking binge and began to argue. Her "husband" (apparently this was not a legal marriage but this is how she referred to him) was almost 20 years older than Roberta. The arguing intensified and turned into a physical confrontation. Roberta beat the man without mercy. After being hospitalized for his injuries, he was admitted to a nursing home where he remained in a vegetative state. Roberta claimed to have no memory of the events of the evening and frequently asked when her husband could come see her. When she was told of his condition and how it occurred, she was extremely upset and continued to deny any knowledge of what happened.

Roberta eventually became competent to stand trial and was found guilty but mentally ill. She served her minimum sentence in the forensic unit and was then transferred to the civil section of the hospital for continued treatment.

An interesting side note of this story is that Roberta's "husband" passed away while in the nursing home and she was the beneficiary of his life insurance policy. It was at first thought she would be unable to claim this money due to being the person who inflicted the injuries on the man. However, it was determined that he died of heart failure and not from any of the injuries inflicted by Roberta, so she was able to collect the money. What irony.

MEET: Freddie

Freddie was a middle-aged male of short stature. He had a very raspy voice and was difficult to understand. He was being treated in the civil section of the hospital for his mental illness and would cycle between improving and relapsing. Freddie's brother was also mentally ill but appeared to fare better and was able to reside in the community. This upset Freddie as he wanted to live with his brother but was too unstable to be released. He would alternate between anger and sadness and really had little insight into his illness.

Freddie did become stable enough to earn privileges to go out on the grounds of the hospital unsupervised for up to 2 hours a day and eventually he earned the privilege to go off grounds unsupervised for up to 2 hours every day. There was a little Mom & Pop store within walking distance that many of the patients would frequent when out on the privilege time.

Apparently, one day, Freddie walked into an open door of one of the houses in the neighborhood near the hospital. There he encountered a young girl and he asked her if she wanted to have sex with him. The police were notified and Freddie was arrested. I am uncertain what charges were filed and which ones he was found guilty of, but he was sentenced to do time in a state prison. I honestly don't know if Freddie would have actually had sex with this young girl. I think he actually craved being close to someone more than having sex.

At the time, I was working in the Activities Department of a state prison. Due to my experiences with mentally ill and mentally retarded individuals, one of my assignments was to provide activities to the inmates in the Special Needs Unit at the prison. This is where prisoners with severe mental illness are housed. One day I arrived on the unit to discover Freddie had been assigned there until arrangements could be made to have him transferred to another state prison for classification. He was locked in his cell 23 hours a day. I spoke to him frequently as he remembered me from when I worked at the hospital, and he showed no understanding of his legal situation. His only concern was when he could get some cigarettes and have some coffee.

Several of the Correctional Officers found Freddie's charges particularly offensive and let him know how they felt about what he had done. This was unprofessional on their part, but it happens. There are many good officers who work well with the mentally ill prisoners, but there are also those who should not be assigned to that unit. This is one of the flaws in the system that I feel needs to be addressed.

Freddie was transferred for classification within a few days and I never heard anymore about him. I am assuming he was sent to the prison that is primarily for prisoners with serious mental health issues.

MEET: Alan

Alan was a long time resident of the forensic unit when I first started working there. He had savagely murdered a cab driver and had been found Not Guilty By Reason of Insanity. This means that he would continue to stay in a state hospital until he was deemed to be "cured" by the unit psychiatrist. I truly believe he is one of the most dangerous people I have ever met and I honestly hope he is never released from the forensic unit.

Alan was in his mid thirties, tall and thin, with long unkempt hair. He was the type of person who could emerge from the shower and still appear dirty. Due to being a chain smoker, he had nicotine stained fingertips and long, dirty fingernails. He usually had a scraggly beard and would wear the same clothes day after day unless staff made him change.

Alan was very psychotic and would spend the majority of his time sitting alone in a corner or hallway, chain-smoking self-rolled cigarettes, and talking to himself. He was usually ranting about his legal issues and what he intended to do to the judge who had heard his case once he was released. If engaged in conversation, he would often describe an invention he thought of or how he could run a business better than anyone else since he was smarter, but eventually, the conversation would return to his legal issues and how he was "railroaded" by a corrupt system. He also had a habit of making machine gun noises while ranting about his case. He was one of the most disturbed and disturbing people I've ever encountered.

Alan was difficult to engage in any type of productive activities but would occasionally watch movies, preferring those with any type of violence in them. This would probably give him additional ideas of things to do to his judge.

Although Alan was actively psychotic despite being on medication, he was usually cooperative with staff and perhaps this was the best we could hope for with someone like him. He didn't use profanity in front of female staff and never, to my knowledge attacked a staff person or another patient. Perhaps the medication kept him from acting on the violence he espoused constantly.

MEET: Patty

For me, the most difficult patients to deal with were those diagnosed with borderline personality disorder. These patients are extremely attention seeking and when they don't get their own way they threaten to inflict or actually inflict harm upon themselves. Usually these self inflicted injuries were non-life threatening but could be serious none the less.

Most of the patients I dealt with having borderline personality disorder were female. When things were going their way, they could be very friendly, helpful, and cooperative people. However, if they felt their perceived needs weren't being met, or they became upset with a relative or staff person for not giving them the attention they felt they deserved, all hell could break loose. Often we would be alerted to a patient's intent of self harm by another patient. This was all part of the game. They would tell another patient knowing that patient would alert staff and then they would be brought into the nursing office to talk about whatever was bothering them and most often would be placed on 1:1 supervision to prevent them from carrying out their threat of self harm. It was a difficult situation to deal with. By placing them on 1:1 you were essentially feeding into their manipulative behavior, but if they did indeed harm themselves, the hospital could be faced with a lawsuit.

Patty was one of those who was generally cooperative and even had a paying job as the unit janitor for awhile. However, due to her self-injurious behaviors, she lost her job as she could not be trusted around cleaning supplies. The one episode of self injury I remember most with Patty required her being hospitalized at a local hospital.

Each unit had a refrigerator in the dayroom where patients could keep juice, milk, or other snacks. One day, while performing security rounds, one of the staff noticed the light bulb in the refrigerator was missing. After checking the maintenance work orders to see if it had been removed for some reason and finding no documentation to that effect, a unit search was conducted. Despite the extensive search, no light bulb was found. Later that shift, a patient came to staff and told them Patty had taken the light bulb, broken it into small pieces, and swallowed it. Patty was brought to the nursing station and confronted with the information we had been given. At first she denied doing anything like this, but after a lengthy conversation with staff and the unit psychiatrist she finally admitted she had indeed swallowed the pieces of the glass light bulb. Dragging out the drama is another way people with this disorder get the attention they crave. It doesn't seem to matter whether the attention is negative or positive, as long as it's attention.

Patty was sent to the local hospital, accompanied by forensic staff. By policy, whenever a forensic patient had to leave the building they had to be shackled and accompanied by forensic unit staff. When Patty was admitted to the hospital, the nurses there did not approve of her being shackled to the bed and demanded the shackles be removed. After several phone calls between both hospital administrators, the shackles remained in place. The nurses tended to treat the forensic unit staff as though they were monsters and unfeeling. How could we possibly be treating this young woman like this after what she had gone through? Well, they got their answer the next day.

When a patient is in 4 point restraints there are precautions that must be taken to ensure proper circulation of the extremities. One extremity can be released for a set period of time to allow freedom of movement. When that extremity is re-shackled, another extremity can be released, and so on. Patty's left hand was released from shackles to enable her to eat a bland breakfast the next morning. A short time later, one of the nurses came in to check Patty's vital signs. The nurse couldn't find the (glass) thermometer anywhere. It had been on the nightstand along with other items and now it was gone. As you can imagine, this caused quite a bit of chaos. Patty initially claimed to have no idea where the thermometer was, but again, after lengthy discussion and cajoling, she admitted she had taken the thermometer while her hand was out of the restraint and swallowed it. The nurses immediately changed their opinion of Patty and blamed the forensic staff for not watching her closely enough. From experience I can tell you, if someone has it in their head to do something like this, they will find a way. Staff members are only human and cannot possibly see everything that goes on in an 8 hour shift, even if they are at arm's length from the patient. We can only do our best.

Patty was discharged from the local hospital very quickly after that incident as it was decided she could receive more direct supervision at the forensic unit and her medical condition was no longer a danger.

MEET: Dennis

When I was working at the state hospital for mentally retarded most of the staff in my unit were between the ages of eighteen and twenty-five. We all got along fairly well and some of us socialized outside of work. Dennis was one of those who would often be at various parties or get-togethers. He had just graduated from high school and was one of the nicest guys you could ever meet. He really seemed to enjoy his job and had a good work ethic. The patients all liked him and so did the staff.

Dennis had naturally curly white-blonde hair and was very good looking. In the summer he wouldn't tan, he'd bronze. Good looking and nice, what a combination!

I only worked with Dennis for a year or so before transferring to another state hospital. After that I kept in contact with some of my former co-workers and began to hear disturbing stories about Dennis. People were saying he was getting "weird" and was expressing strange thoughts. Gradually, people stopped hanging around with him as he was becoming so strange. Some people thought he was involved with drugs and that was what was causing his odd behavior.

One day I happened to be in town and saw Dennis. He remembered me and we stopped to talk. It was then he dropped a bombshell on me. He told me he was at a different institution now. When I asked him how he like working there, he replied, "Oh, I'm not working there, I'm a patient there. I'm just out on a pass for the weekend." I was stunned to say the least. I can't even remember what I said to him after that. It turned out that Dennis had been diagnosed with schizophrenia and had required hospitalization. I suppose that's the first time reality hit me and I realized mental illness could happen to anybody. There were no guarantees that a loved one or myself wouldn't suffer from some type of mental disability.

I ran into Dennis off and on a few times after that. He eventually was placed in a group home where he lived with several other men with various mental illnesses. He generally seemed happy and most often would be listening to his radio while walking around town. Seeing him always made me feel sad because I knew what he had been like prior to getting sick and knew he'd never be able to go back to being that person. I hope wherever he is now, Dennis is stabilized and doing well.

MEET: Miss Mamie

Miss Mamie was one of the first patients admitted into the female forensic unit of the hospital where I worked. At the time, she was in her late 70's. She had been a patient in the civil section of the hospital for many years. To look at her and speak to her you would think she was just a sweet grandmother. She went to church services every week and never gave anyone a bit of trouble. She didn't express any delusional thinking and you might actually wonder why she was in the hospital to begin with. While I'm not sure of the circumstances that brought her to the civil section of the hospital, I do know why she was admitted to the forensic unit. Miss Mamie had killed her roommate in the civil section of the hospital. Her reason for doing so was that she was of the belief her roommate was going to kill her so she decided to kill her first. One night she simply smothered her with a pillow. She did not deny doing it and was found guilty but mentally ill. Therefore, she had to be admitted to the forensic unit, where she remained until she passed away in her mid 80's.

A lot of people were concerned for Miss Mamie's safety since she was being placed on a unit with much younger, rougher, women. The truth was, many of these younger women were scared to death of Miss Mamie! They had all heard that she murdered her roommate and no one wanted to share a room with her. Therefore, Miss Mamie was the only patient to have a private room.

It was interesting to watch the dynamics between the younger women and Miss Mamie. Most of them would go out of their way to be polite to her, get her snacks for her so she didn't have to walk too far, and generally kept an eye out for her. A lot of them called her "Grandmom." In turn, she was very kind to them, unless provoked. I remember watching one incident where a younger patient drank a carton of ice tea from the unit refrigerator that Miss Mamie had brought back from the dining room to drink later. When Miss Mamie went to get the ice tea the other patients told her who had taken it and Miss Mamie stormed over to the girl and chewed her out unmercifully. The girl tried to tell her, "I'm sorry, I didn't know it was yours." To which Miss Mamie replied, "Well, you knew you didn't put it in there so you had no business touching it." It was really quite funny to watch this exchange as the younger woman was definitely afraid Miss Mamie was going to hurt her. In fact, before going to bed that night she asked the staff to be sure to watch the door to her room so Miss Mamie didn't sneak in and kill her.

Miss Mamie was generally a quiet, reserved woman but given the opportunity to converse with staff often had very interesting stories about her life prior to being hospitalized. She talked about her "gentleman friend" and her son and various experiences she had in her life as well as the different jobs she held. It was a shame she had to spend the last years of her life in a mental institution with very little contact with those on the outside. I don't remember her ever getting a visit and she would only receive mail on rare occasions. Still, she remained upbeat and would tease the staff and treat them and the other patients like her family. I think she would have been pleased to see how many people, including staff from the civil section of the hospital came to her memorial service and shared stories of times they spent with her throughout the years.

MEET: Sharon

Sharon was one of the most difficult patients we had to deal with on the forensic unit. She was about 40 years old, 5'10" tall and weighed a little over 200 lbs. Sharon was a very intelligent woman and came from a very good family. On good days, she was interesting to talk to, had a good sense of humor, and could be helpful around the unit. Unfortunately, her good days were outnumbered by her bad days.

On bad days, Sharon would appear very delusional in her thinking and often talked of rats living in her stomach. She was also self-abusive and very attention seeking. Some of the staff felt her self-abusive behavior was due to her delusional thinking, others felt it was more for attention. Each episode of self-abusive behavior would lead to Sharon being placed on 1:1 supervision where she had a staff member within arm's length of her at all times, even when she was sleeping. She remained on 1:1 supervision for months at a time as she would express self-abusive thoughts and continue to make attempts to abuse herself despite being under such close supervision. Some of her self-abusive behaviors included burning her nipple with a cigarette, putting a cigarette into her eye, and running full steam into a glass door (specially made for hospitals where the glass was reinforced with wire mesh and would shatter instead of breaking into shards and the bottom half was made of wood). This last incident I personally witnessed and it is an image I cannot get out of my mind to this day. Sharon took off running down a short hallway and slammed head first into the door to the dayroom. When I heard the noise and looked over, all I could see was Sharon's head sticking through the glass pane of the door. In all honesty, she reminded me of a mounted trophy hanging on a wall. Miraculously, her only injury was a scratch on her cheek.

Sharon was extremely manipulative and was very good at playing staff against one another. There were those who sympathized with her and those who resented her attention seeking behaviors. She was very good at getting certain staff to confide in her about personal issues (which is one of the first things we're taught not to do). She knew what she could get away with and with whom. Some staff were lax in their supervision of her because she would complain she was tired of being followed everywhere, including the bathroom and shower. Yet, when they eased up on their supervision, she would perform one of her self-abusive acts. I personally, never trusted her, and would never cut her any slack, which probably saved me a lot of paperwork.

Occasionally, Sharon's behavior would improve to the point where she would be placed on close observation instead of 1:1. This would mean she would only have to be within sight of staff instead of within arm's length. This would last a few days and then she would do something to be placed on 1:1 again. Despite her protests of hating 1:1 supervision, most of us thought she enjoyed it. She was one of the most draining patients I ever had to work with. The 1:1 supervision would be divided into 4 hour shifts because staff couldn't take more than 4 hours of the stress of being with her.

We would often talk about Sharon's attention seeking behavior and predict that some day she would really harm herself either because someone wasn't paying attention or she took her attempt too far. This is exactly what happened to her. Sharon had resolved her legal issues and was moved to the Civil Section of the hospital. She did fairly well and began to earn some privileges like going out with groups, earning time off the unit by herself, etc. She may have felt she was losing the attention she desperately wanted and would continue to make attempts at self harm. Unfortunately for Sharon, her last attempt went unnoticed until it was too late. She was found hanging in a stairwell of one of the buildings.

Whether she was truly suffering from some type of psychosis or whether she had a personality disorder will always be a topic of debate. The staff did everything they could to keep her safe but in the end could not save her from herself.

MEET: David

I first heard about David when I was working in the civil section of the hospital. A friend of mine who worked in the forensic unit told me about this male patient they had who wore lipstick and tried to dress like a female. Don't ask me how he was able to get lipstick on a male forensic unit, but suffice it to say, where there's a will there's a way.

David's legal issues were eventually resolved but he was deemed still in need of in-patient treatment so he was transferred to the civil section. He was a troubled person who frequently had suicidal ideations and it would appear had transgender issues he was trying to deal with. He continued to try to wear make-up whenever he could and now that he was gaining privileges to go on-grounds by himself, he would often trade cigarettes for make-up with the female patients he met. He also wanted to order dresses and other female clothing from catalogs he received in the mail. His treatment team and psychiatrist denied his requests and attempted to prevent him from wearing make-up by putting in his treatment plan that he would refrain from doing so in order to continue to receive increased privileges.

David contacted the hospital's patient advocate and lodged many complaints claiming he was being denied his right to express himself and dress as he felt he should. The psychiatrist refused to budge from his stance saying that if he allowed this behavior it would be harmful to the other patients. He claimed many of them were very sick and living in non-reality based worlds and if David was allowed to dress as a female while living on a male unit, this would only further confuse the other patients.

David continued to protest his treatment but complied with the decisions made. In conversation he would often talk about having a sex change operation and show off various outfits he liked in the catalogs he got. Many people thought he did this more to shock and see what reaction he could get from those he talked to. I don't know if that was true or not. To the best of my knowledge, the hospital had little experience with treating patients with transgender issues. My feeling is they simply tried to dismiss David's feelings and tried to make him "man up."

David eventually was released from the hospital as he had not had any episodes of harming himself or others. I believe he was out of the hospital less than 6 months when we heard that he had committed suicide by jumping in front of a train. We'll never know why he did it, but my feeling is he was a very conflicted individual and in a lot of emotional pain. Sometimes the pain becomes unbearable and you can't take it anymore.

Since almost 20 years have passed since David died, it would be interesting to see if his treatment program would be any different today than it was then since treatment for those with transgender issues has come so far and the rights of those individuals are taken more seriously. I don't know if it would have saved David's life, but in today's society he might not have felt so alone.

MEET: Barbara and John

I have put Barbara and John in the same section of this book since they both suffer from Huntington's Disease.

This is a disease caused by a genetic defect on chromosome #4. The gene is passed on from generation to generation. The most common form of Huntington's is adult-onset where symptoms begin between the ages of thirty and forty. If one of your parents has Huntington's you have a 50% chance of getting the gene for the disease. If you get the gene from one of your parents, you will develop the disease at some point in your life, and can pass it on to your children. Symptoms include abnormal and unusual movements, quick, sudden jerky movements of arms, legs, and other body parts, unsteady gait, behavioral changes including antisocial behavior, hallucinations, paranoia, psychosis, dementia that slowly gets worse, loss of judgment, loss of memory, speech changes, personality changes, and disorientation.

Huntington's is a progressive disability. There is no cure for the disease and no way to stop it from getting worse. Persons with Huntington's usually die within 15-20 years. Some complications of the disease are loss of ability to care for self, loss of ability to interact, injury to self or others, and increased risk of infection. Depression and suicide are common among persons with Huntington's.

Now that you have an understanding of this cruel and debilitating disease let me begin by telling you about Barbara.

Barbara was married and had 3 children. She had a Masters degree in education. Her family was at the upper end of upper middle class. She had a dream life until in her late thirties she began to show symptoms of Huntington's. Eventually she became unable to care for herself and she was placed in the state hospital. She was very delusional and could be very stubborn and difficult to work with. She treated staff as if they were her servants and could be physically combative. On good days, she would be smiling, try to be helpful around the unit, and enjoyed watching travel videos. During one video on Hawaii she became very excited and announced that she had gone to Hawaii on her honeymoon, which proved to be quite accurate. For years she had very little contact with her husband or children. It was later learned that while her husband kept up on the status of her condition he did not want the children to see their Mother in this condition. Once the children were college age, he decided to let them decide for themselves if they wanted to visit Barbara. I recall them visiting the first time and the absolute joy and recognition Barbara had when she saw them. It was both heart-warming and heart-breaking at the same time. Barbara continued to regress due to her disease and was moved to another area of the hospital where she could receive more assistance with her activities of daily life. She had begun to fall frequently and was beginning to have great difficulty swallowing which led to increased precautions for choking. I had no further contact with Barbara after her relocation to another unit, but often thought of her and how horrible it must be to suffer from such a disease.

John was in his fifties when I first met him. He had once worked for the local government and had two sons. John also had Huntington's and had been placed in the state hospital due to his inability to care for himself and continued deterioration. He was wheelchair bound and could no longer talk. He was also at risk for choking due to swallowing difficulties. When I first met John he had a reputation for striking out at other patients and staff. He would frequently get out of his wheelchair and attempt to walk or even crawl when he wanted to use the bathroom. It appeared he knew when he had to go but was unable to do so independently. He also appeared to feel the need to urinate frequently, as often as 3-4 times an hour. During the night this became very problematic as he would attempt to get out of bed and often injured himself doing so. At one point his bed was moved into the day hall so he could be more closely monitored. Despite not being able to communicate, John understood what was being said to him. I made the suggestion to create a communication board that could be placed on the tray that attached to his wheelchair. On the board I put a variety of pictures along with the typed word underneath. I put a picture of a urinal, a bed, a glass of water, cookies, a picture of a person with a thermometer in their mouth to indicate they were sick, a picture of a smiling person and an unhappy person, in order to help John express his needs to the staff. If he needed to go to the bathroom, he would point to the urinal. If he was thirsty he would point to the glass of water. If he didn't feel well, he could point to the picture of the sick person. At first John needed to be reminded to use the board but once he got used to it he seemed to become less frustrated and there were less incidents of him striking out at others. It was my feeling that much of his anxiety and combativeness was due to not being able to express his needs or have them met. I often thought how I would feel if I were in his position. Here was a man who had held a good job, raised a family, and was obviously a proud individual and now he was totally dependent on others, and most of the time women, to do even the smallest thing for him. I think Huntington's is the cruelest disease there is. I can only hope that someday they are able to find a cure for it.

MEET: Debbie

Debbie was a Hispanic girl in her mid-twenties, approximately 5'9" tall, and weighed about 200 lbs. (when she wasn't using drugs). She had been in and out of county and state correctional facilities for years on various charges including robbery, drug sales, prostitution, etc. Debbie was also a Lesbian. She was admitted to the forensic unit at the state hospital several times due to self-injurious behavior. She would cut herself and had many, many scars on her arms. Some of the professionals thought she was suicidal but she denied that. Her explanation for cutting herself was that it relieved all of the stress and anxiety that was inside her. She claimed once she cut herself she actually felt much calmer.

Generally, Debbie was cooperative on the unit. She was even helpful to some of the patients who needed help in their daily activities. She could be very pleasant, interesting, and had a good sense of humor. However, she also had some very dark days. On these days we knew she was going to cut herself no matter how closely we observed her. Where there's a will there's a way. Debbie could become physically combative if she felt threatened and during the years I knew her she injured several staff members.

Debbie was very masculine in her looks and manner. This appeared to intimidate some of the male staff who worked on the unit or who responded to help during incidents. According to Debbie, they would often say things to her to further aggravate the situation and indicate if she wanted to be a guy they would treat her as one. This is unacceptable in a hospital setting and should never be tolerated. Debbie would often complain about these incidents but there were never any witnesses to corroborate her accusations. I personally have no doubt she was telling the truth as those she would accuse were exactly the type of men who would do such a thing.

Debbie's cutting was due to a personality disorder and medications don't seem to help with that. She could receive medication to reduce her anxiety, but due to her history of drug abuse the psychiatrists were hesitant to give her anything too strong or that could be addictive. Therefore, I would imagine that she is bound to continue to spend time in and out of psychiatric units, and quite possibly correctional facilities the rest of her life.

MEET: Stevie

Stevie was one of the funniest people I've ever met. He was a small, slight man who had an effeminate manner (although I don't know if he was Gay or not). He came to the forensic unit from one of the local county jails due mainly to being a disruption and receiving threats from the other inmates. I think many years of drug use had a part in Stevie's mental illness. He appeared to be a child of the 60's and I can almost picture him stoned out of his mind at Woodstock. I'm not sure what his psychiatric diagnosis was but I would imagine it had to do with some type of personality disorder. Once again, because of his effeminate manner, many of the male staff would shun him and would make jokes about him amongst themselves. Stevie knew this was happening but it didn't bother him one bit. In fact, at times it seemed he would act even more effeminate to watch their discomfort level rise. I would often play cards or Scrabble with Stevie and others during the evening. As I said, he was one of the funniest, most entertaining people I ever met. He had story after story to tell and even the other patients enjoyed his humor . . . most of the time. Stevie was smart enough to know which patients didn't like him and could cause him harm and stayed away from them. He was cooperative and never caused trouble on the unit, except for once. One day when I came on duty, Stevie was in the locked side room (a room used to separate him from others for his or their protection). I couldn't believe it! What could he have possibly done that they locked him up? During shift report we found out that Stevie had grabbed the dayshift nurse's butt. Well, it was all most of us could do not to burst out laughing. This particular nurse was a bitter, miserable woman who wasn't particularly liked by staff and she rarely interacted with the patients other than to give them their medications. After shift report was finished and she had gone for the day, we all started to laugh and figured this had probably been the first time she was grabbed in years! The policy when a patient was in a locked side room was that a sheet was attached to the door that had a variety of questions relating to the patients' condition on it. The patient had to be visually observed and the sheet checked off and signed by a staff person every 15 minutes to ensure the patient was safe. Once the patient was calm and no longer a threat to himself or others he was to be released back out onto the unit. Apparently, Stevie had grabbed the nurse when she was giving out morning medications and had been locked up since that time. The nurse had made a statement to the dayshift staff that Stevie wouldn't come out on their shift. Several of us went back to check on Stevie figuring we would be able to let him out as soon as the nurse was gone for the day, and it had been an isolated incident. When we opened the door to talk to him and assess his mood I told him we would like to let him out but I wanted to know what had possessed him to do such a thing. I will never forget his answer. He said, "I don't know what came over me! I'm so ashamed. I must've been out of my mind to grab *her*! I think I better stay in here a little while longer to repent." That was just the sense of humor Stevie had. We couldn't help but laugh and told him he could repent just as well out in the day hall, he'd been locked up long enough.

MEET: Jerry

Jerry was eighteen years old when he was admitted to the forensic unit of the state hospital. He was a high school dropout who had served very briefly in the U.S. Army. He was discharged when it became apparent he had psychiatric issues. After returning to his parents' home he became disruptive, belligerent, and prone to fits of rage. His mother became fearful of him and worried about the safety of his younger sister. He was told he could no longer live with the family. Jerry continued to show up at their home and the parents finally had him arrested for trespassing. This was done more to have him receive the help he needed than to actually punish him.

When he was admitted to the forensic unit he appeared angry, but cooperative with staff. He had no insight into his behavior and seemed to only focus on the fact that he had been in the Army (albeit for less than a month). He would brag about being a veteran but his youthful appearance made many suspicious of his claims. Many of the other patients thought he was simply delusional. He tried to befriend some of the older patients as the younger ones would often tease him about getting kicked out of the military and taunt him for being overweight.

In the beginning he had most of his daily contact with the staff on the unit. I discovered he enjoyed playing board games and during the early evening hours we would often play Scrabble, cards, or other games available. This also gave me an opportunity to talk with him on a 1:1 level and he eventually let his guard down and discussed some of his issues. During one of our talks he indicated he regretted quitting school. Since he was eighteen, he was eligible to be included in the school program run at the hospital. Teachers were on the grounds to work with any patients twenty-one and under. Those under eighteen had to attend classes but those over eighteen could attend voluntarily. I spoke with the Treatment Team about having Jerry placed into the GED program and he was provided with a teacher who would come to the forensic unit to work with him twice a week. Jerry did very well with his classes and his self confidence began to improve. He would often ask me to help him with his homework in the evening and he became determined to receive his GED so he could continue on to college. During this time Jerry also received medication and therapy to help him with his emotional issues and this proved to be helping him a great deal as well. He became friendlier, smiled more, and began to diet and exercise in the gym in order to lose weight. His mother began to visit and was very happy with the changes she saw. She decided if Jerry continued to do well he could return to the family home after his commitment at the hospital was up.

Jerry was determined to take his GED test before leaving the hospital and spent most of his free time studying. In the evenings, if I was available he would ask me to help him with his studies. For the record, I will say right now, I am glad I wasn't the one having to take the test! The information you need to know is incredible and I had been out of school for many years. I kept telling Jerry, "Rather you than me!"

Jerry took his GED test and then the waiting began for the results. This was a particularly nerve-wracking time for him as not only was he waiting for his test results, but he was approaching the end of his commitment and preparing to leave the hospital. He claimed he wasn't nervous about returning home and felt he could remain in control with the help of his medication and additional out-patient therapy, but I knew he was scared. There was a lot going on at this time and he was still very young. I worried what would happen if he didn't pass his GED. Would that destroy the self-esteem he had built up, would it lead to him giving up, would he react in a negative manner and have his commitment extended? These were all concerns the entire Treatment Team had and would just have to wait to find out.

One day as I arrived on the unit at the beginning of my shift, Jerry approached me smiling broadly. He had gotten the results of his test and had passed! He was so happy and we were happy for him. It looked like things were going to work out for this young man.

The night before Jerry went home he came to me and handed me a xeroxed copy of his GED. He said he wanted me to have it since I had spent so much time helping him. I can't begin to tell you what that meant to me.

I never heard any more about Jerry after he left the hospital. I can only hope he continued to do well and is leading a happy and productive life.

MEET: Bill

Bill definitely appeared to be the type of guy your mother always told you to stay away from. He belonged to a motorcycle gang and was heavily involved in drugs. He was admitted to the forensic unit after trying to commit suicide in jail after being found guilty of murdering his girlfriend

Bill was severely depressed over the death of his girlfriend and the fact that he had killed her. Apparently he had been using drugs quite heavily and one night began having hallucinations. He would never describe these hallucinations but he got his gun and began shooting, killing his girlfriend, although at the time he did not realize it was her. When Bill finally came down from the drugs and realized what he had done, he was horrified. Eventually he tried to hang himself in his jail cell. As he explained, "I believe in an eye for an eye. I took a life, so mine should be taken." He admitted to the crime and asked the judge to sentence him to the death penalty. His lawyer maintained that he had to be mentally unbalanced to ask for the death penalty and the judge agreed. He was sentenced to 20-40 years in the state prison system. He continued to express suicidal ideations and was admitted to the forensic unit for treatment.

Despite Bill's scraggly appearance and history, he was actually a model patient. He was cooperative with staff and eventually earned a job as the unit janitor (a coveted paying position). He was compassionate toward the other patients and would often help out those who were actively psychotic or intellectually impaired. He was very much a favorite among the staff and would spend most evening's playing cards with staff and other patients. His treatment consisted of medication for the depression and therapy sessions. Occasionally Bill would mention he was still having thoughts of suicide and had to be placed on 1:1 supervision for his own safety. These thoughts eventually became less and less, and after approximately two years, Bill was transferred to the state prison system where he continued to serve his time.

I ran into Bill during my first week working at the local state correctional facility. He looked pretty much the same, just older. He said he was doing well and that his brother visited him frequently. He has a job in one of the shops at the prison and appears to be well like by his co-workers and supervisor. He has almost completed his minimum sentence but has not yet seen the Parole Board. Given the situation at this time with violent offenders being paroled, I would assume he would not be granted parole for another few years. If and when he is paroled, I think Bill will do well in the community. He has job skills and a supportive family which are key factors in anyone's success.

MEET: Elizabeth

Elizabeth was admitted to the forensic unit of the hospital due to impulse control problems which got her into fights and charged with assault. She was a very pretty woman in her late twenties and had a combination of Black and Puerto Rican ethnicity. Elizabeth had mental issues in addition to being mildly mentally retarded. She also had hearing loss in one ear and frequently would use this as an excuse for not following instructions or doing what was asked of her.

The main focus of her treatment was to work on her impulse control so that she would develop better coping skills and be able to succeed in the community. Her treatment took on a new dimension however, when one evening she complained of severe stomach pains and had to be taken to an outside hospital for emergency treatment. Ex-rays showed a variety of foreign objects in Elizabeth's stomach and she had to be operated on immediately. Some of the items found in her stomach were: a toothbrush, tube of toothpaste, paper clips, a tampon, buttons, and other small items not meant to be ingested. The term for this behavior is pica, the eating of non-edible items. The staff at the forensic unit were amazed that anyone could ingest these items and realized Elizabeth must have no gag reflex at all. The outside hospital sent her back to the forensic unit after her medical problems were taken care of. For a time, she was placed on 1:1 observation to prevent any further ingestion of foreign matter and then this was reduced to close observation. Eventually, Elizabeth once again began to complain of stomach pains and was returned to the outside hospital for emergency treatment. Once again, it was discovered she had a belly full of paper clips, buttons, various items from arts and crafts group, etc. After her return to the forensic unit, Elizabeth was placed on 1:1 observation and she had large mitts placed on each hand to prevent her from being able to pick up objects that she could ingest. She needed to be on 1:1 observation for her safety, since wearing these mitts also prevented her from being able to protect herself in the event of a fall or attack by another patient.

A treatment plan was written with the goals of eliminating the pica behavior however, this was no easy feat. Despite wearing the mitts and being on 1:1 observation, Elizabeth continued to manage to ingest items that were non-edible. She had to return to the outside hospital for a third time and that hospital began to complain that the forensic unit was not caring for Elizabeth properly. A battle ensued between the forensic unit staff, the treating psychiatrist, Administration, and the outside hospital. It was decided that making Elizabeth wear the mitts or any other type of hand restraints was against her patient rights so the practice was immediately discontinued. She remained on 1:1 observation and her treatment plan was revised multiple times to incorporate short term goals where she would be rewarded for going through set time periods without ingesting foreign matter. She began to show signs of compliance and eventually she was downgraded to close observation. Staff complimented her on her cooperation with her treatment and it was planned that her close observation would soon be discontinued and she would be able to work toward other privileges. Unfortunately, it was discovered that while Elizabeth was complying with her treatment plan and not eating non-edible items, she was sticking small items such as pins, buttons, pencil erasers, etc. in her nose and ears. A new treatment plan had to be written to incorporate this new behavior. Apparently, she enjoyed the attention she received when on 1:1 observation and when her observation level began to drop she found a new way to get the attention she craved. With a new treatment plan in place with many short-term goals put in to reward her positive behavior, Elizabeth eventually stopped the unwanted behaviors. After her legal issues were resolved, she was transferred into the civil unit of the hospital where she began to earn various privileges up to and including being able to go out onto the grounds without supervision. I don't know if she ever resumed the pica behavior, but would imagine she may have from time to time when she wanted attention.

MEET: Richard

Richard was in his first year of college when he became withdrawn, delusional, disorganized, and began to hear voices. He was diagnosed with schizophrenia and his family placed him in the state hospital. I always found this to be interesting as Richard's father was a psychiatrist at a different state hospital. Apparently he had tried to medicate his son but the symptoms continued and Richard became too much for his mother to care for and his father seemed to look at him as an embarrassment. They never visited or made any effort to find out how he was doing.

Apparently, Richard had been a fairly normal child and did well in school. He enjoyed sports and played baseball throughout his school years. It's hard to say if any particular event caused his psychotic break but this is the general age group when schizophrenia occurs.

Richard was in his mid-thirties and was extremely quiet. He would give one word answers to questions but was able to speak in a complete sentence if he had to. He was extremely disorganized and had trouble following simple instructions, although he tried to do what was asked of him. He would frequently chuckle to himself and often seemed to be responding to internal stimuli. Richard had one other symptom that is seen in many schizophrenics. He had polydipsia, which is the excess drinking of water (or other fluids) to the point of water intoxication. This is an extremely dangerous condition as the patient drinks so much that he/she can throw their electrolytes off balance and in extreme cases this can cause death. Richard was unable to stop himself from drinking massive quantities of water during waking hours. He could gain as much as 12 lbs. in a day all from water weight. Patients with polydipsia have to be monitored very closely. If left unsupervised they will frequently be found drinking water from a water fountain, sink, or even a toilet if that's all that's available. In a hospital setting a unit for patients with polydipsia is often set up so that water can be shut off to sinks and fountains to help eliminate this behavior but realistically, once the patient is sent to another unit or earns privileges of time unsupervised, or is discharged from the hospital they continue the behavior.

Richard tried to be cooperative with his treatment program, but had no insight into his illness and didn't understand why he was being asked to complete certain tasks, take care of his personal hygiene, or refrain from excessive fluid intake. While

Richard was not physically combative, many patients who have polydipsia can become combative when their fluid intake is limited.

Richard enjoyed going on trips away from the hospital such as going bowling, to the movies, or just going for van rides. Plans were in progress for Richard to move into a community living arrangement but unfortunately he passed away from cancer prior to this happening.

MEET: Jim

Jim's story is similar to Richard's in that he seemed to have a fairly normal childhood but became ill during his late teens. Jim was diagnosed with schizophrenia and also had polydipsia. His family managed to keep him at home until both parents passed away and his brother could not provide the care and supervision Jim required. He was then admitted to the state hospital.

Jim was in his late twenties and had a boyish innocence about him. He frequently talked about times spent with his family at the shore working on their boat. His goal in life was to live at the shore and get a job working on boats and in his off time go sailing and fishing. He spoke about this often.

Jim's polydipsia was severe and he would become very psychotic and delusional after ingesting large amounts of water. He would actively respond to internal stimuli and often become verbally combative with the voices he was hearing as well as the staff on the unit. He had absolutely no insight into his illness and could not understand why he had to be in the hospital. Although he knew his treatment plan goals and objectives, he was not interested in working on them. This is not unusual for schizophrenic patients.

Jim enjoyed participating in activities but needed a great deal of prompting to complete tasks as he had difficulty focusing his attention on tasks due to the interference of internal stimuli. He could often be seen talking to or even arguing with the voices he was hearing, laughing inappropriately, or during group sessions talking about topics that weren't being discussed.

He was still hospitalized when I left my employment at the hospital.

MEET: Joan

The staff working on the female forensic unit knew we would be getting Joan as a patient. We had all seen the many news reports and knew this woman would not be safe in a county correctional facility. She was obviously mentally ill and the forensic unit would be able to afford her treatment as well as increased safety.

Joan was a highly educated woman in her mid-thirties. Her husband had several medical problems that he was receiving treatment for and this was one stressor in her life. Joan began to have some medical issues of her own and went to between twelve and fifteen doctors, none of which were able to find anything wrong with her. Joan became convinced she and her husband were going to die. At the time they had two young children and Joan was extremely worried about what would happen to the children when she and her husband died. Unfortunately, she decided that it would be best for the children if they died first. In her mind, she felt this way they would remain together and not have to suffer. Joan proceeded to drown her children in the bathtub of the family home. Her husband found the children when he came home from work.

While the various physicians Joan went to for help for her medical complaints found nothing wrong, not one of them suggested to her that she consult a psychiatrist. If she had done so, perhaps the tragedy could have been avoided, but no one will ever know for sure.

When Joan came to the forensic unit, she was very quiet, had an almost dazed look about her, and was placed on suicide precautions. She was placed on psychotropic medications and in time began to become more like what she had probably been like before her illness took over. Joan was a very bright woman and very much aware of what she had done and that she would probably remain in prison for the rest of her life. Her husband would visit weekly and this could be gut-wrenching to witness. At times he would be angry, crying, accusing her of ruining their family. He once brought pictures of the children and when she became hysterical he told her she should have to see them because he has to look at them every day. Fortunately, her husband began treatment for the trauma that had occurred and his psychiatrist worked in conjunction with the forensic unit psychiatrist to ensure both would be closely monitored. At first it was felt that the husband's visits were detrimental to Joan's treatment, but she pleaded to be able to see him. She felt she deserved whatever he had to say. She also felt sorry for him as she had ruined his life and he had no one to talk to. Despite everything that had happened, it was obvious Joan's husband still loved her, but could not fathom what she had done, and wasn't sure how to continue on with his life.

Once Joan was deemed to be competent to stand trial, it went pretty much the way everyone expected. She was found guilty but mentally ill. This meant she would stay at the forensic hospital until her mental illness was cured and then she would go to a state prison for women.

Joan spent several years in the forensic unit and was a model patient. She really was one of the favorites among the staff and the other patients liked her as well. When it came time for her to be transferred to the state prison, it was difficult as the staff knew she would face a tough road there. From everything we have heard, she managed to adjust well. Her husband sold their home so that he could buy a place closer to the prison in order to be able to visit her on a regular basis.

This was one of the saddest cases I've ever seen. It shows that mental illness doesn't care if you're intelligent or ignorant, wealthy or poor. Anyone can have a psychotic break and it can ruin not only their life, but the lives of those closest to them.

MEET: Sarah

Sarah came to the forensic unit from the state women's prison due to being depressed and suicidal. She was very petite and only twenty years old. She had recently begun serving a sentence for killing her husband. While I am not sure exactly what crime Sarah was found guilty of (possibly voluntary manslaughter), I believe she received a sentence of 10-20 years. She would still be a young woman when released and could hopefully move on with her life.

Sarah was from a small town and probably had never ventured further than the Jersey shore. She became pregnant, got married, and had her first child when she was sixteen. By the time she was twenty, she had three children.

Sarah's life revolved around her children. There is no doubt she was a good mother. Unfortunately, her husband, while seemingly a good father to his children, was abusive to his wife. He would physically abuse her without warning and often in front of the children. Sarah was more concerned about the children seeing this behavior than she was about the actual abuse. She often threatened to leave her husband but he told her he would make sure she would never see the children again so she stayed.

One evening as Sarah was making dinner, her husband came home and began to taunt her and the taunting turned physical. The children were within view of all of this and it seems something in Sarah simply snapped. She reached for the closest thing she could find, which turned out to be a steak knife, and stabbed her husband to death. She said she was "just tired of him doing this to me in front of the children all of the time."

Sarah admitted her guilt and knew she would have to serve prison time. Her parents told her they would take her children into their home and raise them until she was released from prison. They also promised to bring them to see her when they could. In this aspect, Sarah was lucky, her children would continue to be in a loving home and she would be able to see them.

Although Sarah knew her children were in good hands she became very depressed whenever she thought about how she had killed her husband. She especially regretted doing it in front of the children and realized they may have psychological issues in the future. While Sarah was generally a quiet person, she became more withdrawn and would often become tearful when discussing her situation. She became upset whenever she thought about taking the children' father away from them and often stated she probably deserved the way he treated her. At the prison, they began to fear that Sarah might attempt suicide so she was sent to the forensic unit at the hospital for treatment.

Sarah received intense therapy and soon began to show signs of improvement. She stayed in the forensic unit for approximately 6 months and then returned to the state prison. We frequently heard reports that she was doing well and was considered a model inmate. Hopefully she was paroled after her minimum sentence was served and she was able to return home to her parents and children.

This is an example of how quickly a person's life can be changed by one impulsive act. However, at the time, this was the only way Sarah could see getting her children and herself out of what seemed to be an impossible situation.

Unfortunately, Sarah's story is not unusual. Instead of seeking help, many women stay in abusive relationships often for a variety of reasons. They may be afraid for their lives or the lives of their children, they may feel they deserve the abuse, they may not know of anywhere safe to go, or they may believe that it won't happen again. My advice to anyone involved in an abusive situation is to get help through any of the various support groups that are available. Check your telephone book, ask your clergy or doctor, and do what you have to do to keep yourself safe. Taking matters into your own hands will only make a bad situation much worse.

MEET: Rosie

Rosie had been serving a state prison sentence for robbery when she was transferred to the forensic unit of the state hospital due to anorexia and bulimia. She was approximately 5'6" tall and rail thin. She may have weighed around 100 lbs. What struck me most about her appearance was the pallor of her skin. She appeared to have a greenish tint to her.

Rosie was immediately put on 1:1 supervision and her treatment plan was initially for her not to lose any more weight and then to add a certain amount of weight each week. It may have been as little as one-half pound but with people like Rosie you might as well be asking them to gain 100 lbs.

The staff on the unit quickly became aware of how clever patients suffering from these disorders can be. They may appear to eat but are quite sleight of hand. If watched when they eat, they will take the next available moment to vomit (and can come up with interesting places to hide the evidence). Rosie was being weighed daily and at first seemed to be complying with her treatment by not losing weight. It was then discovered that she was putting heavy objects in her pockets to make it look like she hadn't lost weight when indeed she had. The next step was to weigh her each day while she was completely nude. This infuriated her to no end and she would often refuse to eat anything. She required frequent blood work to monitor her electrolytes and several times came very close to having to be hospitalized at the local hospital in order to be fed intravenously. This seemed to frighten her and she would become compliant for a short period of time but then resort to her previous behavior.

Rosie was a very difficult patient to deal with as the forensic unit was not set up for patients with eating disorders. We had twenty five other patients with various forms of mental illness, some of them very psychotic and in need of close supervision and assistance. It was hard for the staff to have much empathy for Rosie when her behavior appeared to be in her control. It was an endless cycle of compliance and non-compliance. She appeared to have borderline personality disorder as well and she was very good at manipulating staff. She was without a doubt, one of the most difficult patients we had to deal with.

Staff on the unit became very frustrated as every time Rosie lost weight, they were held responsible and told they weren't following the psychiatrist's orders and watching her as they should. The staff tried to explain there were other patients on the unit that needed attention and the unit was not set up to deal with this type of disorder but the protests fell on deaf ears since the psychiatrist found Rosie to be a "very interesting patient."

Rosie was still in the forensic unit when I left. While her legal issues may have been long ago resolved, I doubt she ever regained her physical health. In all honesty, I would suspect she may no longer be alive. She had a history of drug abuse and prostitution. With her immune system compromised by her anorexia and bulimia she would be a prime candidate for TB, HIV infection or other sexually transmitted diseases that she probably wouldn't get treatment for.

MEET: Paul

When I first saw Paul I could not imagine why he was in a state hospital. He was in his mid-twenties, well groomed, and appeared in touch with reality. I found out that Paul had been in the hospital for several months due to being bi-polar (formally called manic-depressive). When he was first admitted to the hospital he was in an extremely depressive state. Apparently during his prior manic episode he had spent thousands of dollars, maxed out all of his credit, but admittedly, had the time of his life. Unfortunately, this all came crashing down around him when the bills started coming in and he had no money to pay them. His family had been through periods like this with him before and would no longer pay his bills. They were angry with him for his lack of self control and did not realize at the time that he couldn't help what he was doing. Paul had a sister he was very close to and it was through her encouragement that he sought psychiatric help. Paul was prescribed lithium for his condition. This medication is very helpful in the treatment of bi-polar patients. The downside is that it requires extensive blood work to ensure the medication is at the proper levels. This is one reason many patients on lithium stop taking it after awhile, they do not like having to have the blood work done on a monthly or even less basis. Many patients report they feel fine and no longer need to take the medication and that is when the trouble begins all over again. Once the medication is out of their system, the highs and lows begin again.

Paul appeared to have good insight into his illness and when he was discharged from the hospital went to live with his sister. Whether or not he continued to comply with his medication routine, I don't know. Paul is one patient I would think had a good chance of staying compliant especially since he had a supportive family member to keep an eye on him. I'm sure if he began to show signs of becoming manic or depressed his sister would notify his doctor.

MEET: Tony

Tony was in the forensic unit of the state hospital when I first met him. He was about nineteen years old and was mildly retarded in addition to having a personality disorder. He was extremely attention seeking and would often threaten to harm himself in order to be placed on 1:1 observation. Another one of his tactics was to threaten or actually attack one of the bigger, stronger patients so that that patient would hit him. Then Tony would have to be placed on 1:1 for his own protection. Tony was the type of patient that simply could not let you have a peaceful shift. He had to be observed constantly even when he wasn't officially on any type of watch.

One evening right before the change of shift at 11:00 p.m. Tony came to the office and reported that another patient had raped him in the dorm. All reports of this nature have to be taken seriously so staff began the procedures that are set in place when something like this happens. Tony and the other patient had to be put on close observation and they had to bring their beds (Including the linens on them) into the dayhall area. State police had to be contacted, incident reports had to be written, the Superintendent had to be notified, and Security had to be notified. All staff on duty had to remain on duty as Tony had to be escorted to the local hospital to be examined. After approximately three hours of turmoil, Tony finally admitted the other patient had not raped him and that he had made it all up for attention.

Tony eventually ended up being sent to another forensic unit in the state where treatment was more intense. I don't think it helped him too much though since the last time I saw him he was in one of the special needs units of a state prison.

Tony appeared to be getting more deviant in his behavior. His sister met with the Unit Social Worker and showed him several letters she had received from Tony. In these letters, Tony described in vivid detail what he planned to do to her sexually once he was released from jail. These were some of the most disgusting, vile letters I have ever seen. It was no wonder his sister was fearful that he would one day be released. The last I had heard of Tony, he had once again been transferred to the forensic unit of another state hospital for more intensive treatment.

MEET: Ginny

Ginny was admitted to the female forensic unit on charges of vagrancy and stealing small items out of stores. I think this was another case where the police pressed charges in order for her to receive the psychiatric treatment she needed.

Ginny was a street person and was approximately in her mid 40's. She had salt and pepper hair and was a light skinned Black woman with freckles over the bridge of her nose. Generally, she was cooperative with staff except on two occasions. She didn't want to take her medication and she refused to shower. The nurse received a doctor's order to give Ginny and injection if she refused to take her meds orally. That took care of that problem and only required one injection before Ginny decided taking the meds wasn't such a bad idea. The problem of showering was another issue altogether.

The staff on the unit had to have the psychiatrist write an order that gave us permission to physically put Ginny in the shower and wash her body and hair on an every other day basis until she became compliant. This was not a pleasant task. I happened to be there the first night we had to shower Ginny. At first Ginny attempted to fight us on the way to the shower room but realized there were far more of us than there was of her so she became somewhat cooperative but would not wash herself. We had to actually go into the shower with her (wearing gowns over our clothing and several pairs of rubber gloves) and scrub her down. It had probably been months since she had showered and the stench was horrible. Worse yet was when the water hit her hair! It was truly a horrible smell that came from her. We shampooed her hair about three times to get all of the dirt out of it and scrubbed her down from head to foot. The whole time Ginny was hollering about us touching her in her "female parts" and that we had no right to do that. We told her if she would do it herself we wouldn't have to and would very much prefer it that way. After her shower we gave her a clean nightgown, sock, slippers, and bathrobe which she seemed to appreciate. We had to go through this ritual about three times before Ginny finally started showering herself. We still had to go into her dorm and take her dirty clothes and replace them with clean ones as Ginny saw no need to ever wash her clothes.

Ginny eventually became compliant with most of the unit rules and would often sit and talk with staff or watch TV with the other patients in the evening. One evening I sat down next to her to talk with her for awhile and she asked me if I wanted some chicken. I found this to be a very strange question and was curious as to what she would do if I said yes. So, I told her since I hadn't gone to dinner yet, that would be nice. Lo and behold, she pulled several pieces of chicken from out of her bra! It was all I could do to keep a straight face. She had stored it there from lunch and I suppose was planning on having a mid-night snack. I guess you just can't take the street out of some people.

MEET: Matthew

Matthew was brought to the forensic unit of the state hospital due to being uncontrollable in the county jail. Basically, he was creating such a commotion; the other prisoners were threatening to beat him up. He was constantly ranting and raving; would initiate arguments with the other prisoners and talked non-stop day and night even if no one was listening. The county jail officials were afraid he would get hurt and they suspected mental health issues so he was sent to the forensic unit.

Matthew was a short Black man in his mid to late sixties. He was bald except for a fringe of white hair around his head and had a full white beard. He was a small man, but certainly made up for his size by making his presence known!

Matthew's charges were minor and once again it appeared the police charged him in order to get him the mental health evaluation and help he needed.

Matthew had an opinion on everything and would share it with anyone within ear shot. He blamed most of his troubles on the White people but yet he was friendly toward White patients and staff. He would go on for hours about his various opinions but generally was cooperative with staff. While many of his ideas may have seemed paranoid, you have to remember the time-frame Matthew grew up in. His family was from the South and many of them had been slaves. I suppose this is where Matthew learned his dislike of White people. Whenever he would go on one of his rants about White people and I was on duty, he would look at me and say, "Now I don't mean you Miss Patricia." I actually enjoyed Matthew and as his medication began to work and he calmed down, he would often sit with me in the evening and talk about events in his life. Some of his more interesting stories dealt with when he worked as a porter on the railroads. He really had led an interesting life.

You must remember, Matthew was hospitalized back in the early to mid 1980's. In retrospect, I think he was showing signs of Alzheimer's but at that time we weren't as aware of that disease as we are now. Matthew could tell you stories about his childhood, travels, family, etc. but had difficulty following simple instructions. Eventually, we had to make him bring his bed into the day room each night to sleep because the other patients couldn't get any rest due to his constant rambling.

He was as cooperative as he could be given his confusion at times. Frequently he forgot where the bathroom was and would urinate in the corner of the day room, much to the distress of the other patients and staff. His personal hygiene was fair but he frequently needed reminders to change his clothes and do his laundry. Staff would help him with his laundry as he could not remember how to use the washing machine and dryer.

Matthew always reminded me of somebody's grandfather. The one who had a twinkle in his eye, was mischievous, but pretty much harmless. I think if he had entered the system after more was known about Alzheimer's, his treatment would have been different. Perhaps the medications would have been the same but his treatment plan would have included more assistance with his activities of daily living skills and attempts to limit his outbursts.

I don't know what ever happened to Matthew, but I must say I enjoyed meeting him and listening to some of his stories. Many people don't want to be bothered listening to the stories of the elderly or simply don't have time with everything else they need to do, but I found that whenever I was able to listen to not only Matthew but some of the other older patients I always learned something.

MEET: Mrs. Michael Jackson

Chantelle came to the forensic unit from one of the local county jails. Her initial charges were defiant trespass and resisting arrest. During her time in the county jail, Chantelle became problematic as her delusions gave the other prisoners fuel to tease and torment her, which would then result in assaultive behavior.

Chantelle presented herself very well. She had been a secretary at a local firm, lived on her own, and seemed to be doing well. At one point, she sued a large corporation in the Philadelphia area when she fell and broke her leg on a damaged sidewalk in front of their building. From what we were told, she received $50,000 from the lawsuit.

Chantelle firmly believed that she was married to Michael Jackson. She did not insist on being called Mrs. Jackson or Chantelle Jackson, but she would tell everyone that she was his wife. On one occasion when he was on a television special she sat front row in the day room to watch it and was seen smiling and talking to him through the television. Of course, some of the other patients would taunt her and tell her she was not married to Michael Jackson, but Chantelle would simply dismiss this as them being jealous.

Chantelle got into the habit of sending home care packages for Michael. She would send out boxes through the unit mail addressed to him at her former apartment address. Technically, we as staff were not allowed to open incoming or outgoing patient mail. However, we received a complaint from her former apartment building manager that there were boxes of mail addressed to Michael Jackson piling up at her door. The unit psychiatrist told us that this was not our problem and to continue to let the mail go out. Well, we as unit staff, could not see Chantelle having to pay for the postage for these boxes to be sent out knowing that no one would be receiving the packages. We began opening the boxes after she went to bed and were surprised at the items she was mailing out! She was sending "Michael" money ($5 or so from her unit job), cigarettes, peanut butter crackers, towels from our shower room, etc. along with letters. We never read the letters but destroyed them and made sure no one would be able to retrieve them. As for the other items, we would see to it that any cash she attempted to send was put back into her account, we would give her the cigarettes when she ran low, and would put the snack items out with other items in the evening. The towels and other linens were simply put back into the laundry.

Yes, we disobeyed the orders of the unit psychiatrist, but we felt it made much more sense than having her send out items she could use, knowing no one would receive them, or that they would probably be stolen from her apartment door.

Chantelle did not feel she had any type of mental illness and couldn't understand why people did not believe she was Michael Jackson's wife. However, she did agree to take the medication that was prescribed for her. Unfortunately, her delusion appeared to be so deep rooted that none of the medication she was given while I worked with her did much good. Other than believing she was married to Michael Jackson, Chantelle appeared very functional. I'm sure once her legal issues were resolved she would be able to return to the community and live on her own, get a job, and carry on much as she had prior to her scrape with the law.

MEET: Ed

Ed was a Vietnam veteran who had for some unknown reason taken several people hostage in a farmhouse. I am not sure of the events that lead up to this event, but I know when police and the SWAT team attempted to free the hostages at least some were shot and killed by Ed.

Ed never denied his role in the hostage situation or killing some of the hostages. He was admitted to the forensic unit from the county jail where he was awaiting trial because he had attempted suicide.

Ed was very depressed and rarely talked about his situation to anyone other than his psychiatrist and his roommate whom he had become very close to. He was truly a model patient and never gave staff or other patients any problem. He had some good days when we would actually see him smile once in awhile (usually when he and his partner won a game of pinochle). However, most days he would spend most of his time pacing the unit and not interacting with anyone.

On several occasions, Ed attempted to commit suicide on the unit, usually at night when he thought no one would be checking on him. Fortunately, staff go on rounds frequently and check on all the bedrooms and dorm areas throughout the night. Each time Ed was discovered and saved from his attempt.

Eventually, Ed went to trial and was sentenced to life in prison without the possibility of parole. He left the Forensic Unit and went to one of the state prisons. Within six months of being in prison, Ed successfully committed suicide.

According the background information we had on Ed, prior to his service in the Army, he was a fairly happy individual, had a job, and friends in his home town. Many people believe that Ed's life changed drastically due to things he saw and did while serving in Vietnam.

MEET: Joe

I was new to working at this particular state hospital and getting to know the patients on my assigned unit as well as patients from other units who came to evening activities when I first saw Joe. He was of medium build, fair-skinned, and had very dark black hair (obviously dyed). I thought there was something familiar about him, but figured perhaps I just knew him from another hospital that I had worked at.

It wasn't until I heard someone call him by name that I realized where I knew Joe from. We were in the same graduating class at high school. What had thrown me off was that in high school; Joe's hair was very light blonde. Other than that, he looked pretty much the same as he had in school.

I don't remember if Joe and I had any classes together, but we knew each other enough to say hi. I remember him as being quiet, pretty much a loner, and very artistic.

After a few weeks of seeing him off and on at various activities I finally spoke to Joe and introduced myself. He said he thought he recognized me and we spoke very briefly about going to school together,

It seems Joe was another person who suffered from schizophrenia that came on during late adolescence. At the time, even though Joe was in the hospital, he appeared to be doing well and would go home on weekends with his parents. It was hoped that when Joe was well enough he would go to live in a group home in the community. I never found out if this happened as I left the hospital before he did.

I felt very bad when I learned of Joe's illness. He was such a bright and gifted young man when we were in school. It definitely shakes you up when you meet someone you knew prior to their illness in a psychiatric hospital setting. This was similar to how I felt when my former co-worker Dennis told me he was in a psychiatric hospital after we had both worked at a hospital for mentally retarded individuals. You start to wonder, "Why them?" Then you are thankful you still have your mental health.

Final Thoughts

These are just some of the people I have encountered in my thirty four years of working in the mental health and corrections field. There are others I have chosen not to write about as their stories are too disturbing or have already been told repeatedly in the newspapers or on television. I simply wanted to provide a range of the patients I have encountered.

I cannot stress enough the importance of realizing that patients are first and foremost human beings. They could have been your neighbor, a school mate, a relative, or even you. Therefore, please always remember, no matter what atrocities a patient may have committed, they did so because they were sick. You must always treat the patient as a human being

Working with the mentally ill, especially those in the forensic unit, is often difficult. There are days when it seems the entire unit is acting out. I cannot count the number of times I was hit, punched, and spit on by patients, (and these were the females). But, you cannot retaliate. You have to remember that these individuals are mentally ill, and often are not in control of their actions. Of course, there are some patients that use that as an excuse to assault a staff person and know that they will pretty much get away with it. Staff can and sometimes do press charges on patients who assault them but this is discouraged by the administration. It's pretty much an unwritten rule that the patients are sick and not in control of their actions and you knew the risks when you took the job.

As you know, the patients I've written about are the ones who are hospitalized. There are many other people in the community who suffer from various forms of mental illness but are able to function well and lead productive lives often by taking medication and seeing therapists or a psychiatrist. Many who know me aren't aware of this but I have been diagnosed with severe depression and an anxiety disorder. I take my prescribed medication daily and am happy to say that it is working well for me.

If, after reading this book, you think working with the mentally ill is something you would like to do I would suggest contacting a psychiatric hospital in your area and signing on as a volunteer for awhile. They are always looking for volunteers to help with patient events or visit patients who don't receive visitors. This will give you an even better idea if this type of work is for you.

I would also like to urge various community organizations to consider reaching out to anyone in your area who may be struggling with mental illness. Many ex-patients now living in the community feel very alone and would love to have someone invite them to church, visit them occasionally, or simply remember their birthday. Showing kindness will make you feel good and could possibly be a great motivator for the recipient.

www.ingramcontent.com/pod-product-compliance
Lightning Source LLC
Chambersburg PA
CBHW021254280526
45784CB00005B/2375